FERTILITY DIET COOKBOOK FOR WOMEN

"Recipes Packed with Nutrients to Optimize Your Chances of Getting Pregnant"

Allie Nagel

Copyright © 2023 by Allie Nagel

DISCLAIMER

This cookbook is intended to provide general information and recipes. The recipes provided in this cookbook are not intended to replace or be a substitute for medical advice from a physician.

The reader should consult a healthcare professional for any specific medical advice, diagnosis or treatment.

Any specific dietary advice provided in this cookbook is not intended to replace or be a substitute for medical advice from a physician.

The author is not responsible or liable for any adverse effects experienced by readers of this cookbook as a result of following the recipes or dietary advice provided.

The author makes no representations or warranties of any kind (express or implied) as to the accuracy, completeness, reliability or suitability of the recipes provided in this cookbook.

The author disclaims any and all liability for any damages arising out of the use or misuse of the recipes provided in this cookbook.

The reader must also take care to ensure that the recipes provided in this cookbook are prepared and cooked safely. The recipes provided in this cookbook are for informational purposes only and should not be used as a substitute for professional medical advice, diagnosis or treatment.

TABLE OF CONTENTS

INTRODUCTION

Sarah's dream of becoming a mother had always been an integral part of her life. She had pictured herself cradling a little bundle of joy, watching their tiny fingers grasp hers, and feeling the indescribable warmth of a child's love.

However, fate had dealt her a cruel hand infertility had become an uninvited guest in her life.

The journey through infertility was a relentless rollercoaster of emotions that left Sarah feeling broken and defeated. The sting of disappointment each month as she awaited the arrival of her period was a constant reminder of her body's apparent inability to conceive.

 Friends and family members joyfully announced their pregnancies, while Sarah's heart ached with envy, longing for the chance to experience the miracles of motherhood.

Infertility had become a dark cloud that loomed over every aspect of Sarah's life. It impacted her relationships, causing strains and misunderstandings.

The innocent questions of, "When are you having a baby?" transformed into piercing daggers that wounded her soul.

Each baby shower she attended was a painful reminder of what she yearned for but could not have.

Determined not to surrender to despair, Sarah embarked on a quest to find a solution. She spent countless hours researching and consulting with medical professionals, but the answers seemed elusive.

Frustrated by the lack of progress, she stumbled upon a book that would change her life forever.

This book, filled with stories of hope and recovery, highlighted the transformative power of nutrition.

Sarah learned that what she consumed could directly impact her hormonal balance and reproductive health. Intrigued by this revelation, she delved into the world of nutrition, determined to regain control of her body and find a path to motherhood.

Sarah overhauled her diet, bidding farewell to processed foods and embracing whole, nutrientdense ingredients. She incorporated colorful fruits and vegetables, lean proteins, and healthy fats into her meals.

She discovered the healing properties of foods like leafy greens, avocados, and nuts, all of which were packed with essential vitamins and minerals.

As Sarah nourished her body with wholesome foods, she noticed subtle changes within herself.

Her energy levels soared, her mood stabilized, and she regained a sense of empowerment. But the ultimate test was yet to come could these dietary changes truly impact her fertility?

Months passed, and with every passing cycle, Sarah began to notice something extraordinary. The symptoms of hormonal imbalance that had plagued her for years began to fade.

Her menstrual cycle became more regular, and the agonizing cramps that had accompanied it diminished. Hope began to blossom in her heart.

Then, on a fateful day, Sarah's dream came true. Two pink lines appeared on the pregnancy test, ushering in a wave of disbelief, joy, and overwhelming gratitude.

In that moment, she knew that her perseverance and dietary

changes had played a crucial role in her victory over infertility. Sarah's story serves as a powerful testament to the healing potential of simple changes in our daily lives.

It reminds us that sometimes the answers we seek are not found in complex medical interventions but in the basic elements of our existence: the food we consume and the choices we make.

Her journey through infertility taught her the invaluable lesson of resilience, the strength to face adversity headon, and the belief that miracles are possible, even in the face of seemingly insurmountable odds.

Today, as Sarah cradles her precious baby in her arms, she is a living testament to the transformative power of hope, determination, and the profound impact of nutrition on our bodies.

So, to every woman out there facing the challenges of infertility, I implore you to hold onto hope. Embrace the possibility of change, and remember that sometimes the most profound transformations can occur through the simplest of choices.

CHAPTER 1

An Overview on Fertility Diet for Women

A fertility diet is a dietary pattern that is rich in certain nutrients that can help increase the chances of successful conception, and encourage the growth and development of a healthy baby.

Nutrient rich foods can help improve fertility and support a healthy pregnancy.

One of the key components of a fertility diet for women is the consumption of foods that are rich in folate, which can help reduce the risk of neural tube defects in newborns.

These foods include dark leafy greens such as spinach and kale, dark oranges or tangerines, and fortified whole grains such as oatmeal.

Legumes, such as beans, split peas, and lentils, also contain a significant amount of folate.

Other elements that can improve a woman's fertility and support a healthy pregnancy are the consumption of foods containing healthy fats, such as avocados, olives, walnuts, and other nuts. Eating healthy fats can help balance hormones and maintain proper blood flow to the reproductive organs.

Consuming a variety of lean proteins, such as chicken, fish, turkey, eggs, and dairy, can also support fertility health by providing essential vitamins and minerals.

Omega3 fatty acids found in salmon, mackerel, walnuts, and flaxseed are essential for reproductive health and can help reduce inflammation that can lead to infertility.

A fertility diet should also include foods that are rich in antioxidants, such as blueberries, apples, tomatoes, sweet potatoes, and bell peppers.

These foods can help reduce inflammation and protect the body from environmental toxins, which can negatively affect fertility health.

An effective fertility diet should also contain plenty of water. Staying hydrated is essential to promote fertility and protect reproductive health.

Along with a healthy diet, it's important for women to manage stress, get enough rest, and stay active.

20 Benefits of Fertility Diet for Women

1. Balancing hormones: A fertility diet helps to balance a woman's hormones, such as estrogen, progesterone, and testosterone.

2. Reducing inflammation: The diet includes antiinflammatory foods, such as fatty fish and leafy greens that can help reduce inflammation in the body.

3. Increasing fertility: Foods like whole grains, fruits, vegetables, legumes, nuts, and fish, which are included in a fertility diet, can help improve a woman's fertility.

4.Boosting the immune system: A fertility diet includes foods that are rich in vitamins and minerals that support a strong immune system.

5. Improving digestion: Whole grains, fruits, vegetables, legumes, and nuts help improve digestion and reduce digestive symptoms like gas and bloating.

6. Regulating blood sugar levels: A fertility diet regulates blood sugar levels and helps control cravings and improve energy levels.

7. Boosting fertility-friendly nutrients: A fertility diet is rich in fertilityfriendly nutrients like zinc, folate, omega3 fatty acids, and antioxidants, which are essential for fertility and ovulation.

8. Increased energy: A fertility diet can provide the right amount of energy needed for everyday activities.

9. Reducing stress: The foods in a fertility diet, such as omega3 fatty acids, help to reduce the stress hormone cortisol in the body.

10. Preventing conditions like PCOS: A fertility diet helps to prevent conditions like Polycystic Ovarian Syndrome (PCOS) that can affect fertility.

11. Lowering risk of miscarriage: Eating the right foods for fertility can lower the risk of miscarriage and help a woman have a healthy pregnancy.

12. Supporting liver health: A fertility diet supports the liver's role in hormone production and helps promote healthy pregnancy.

13. Increasing libido: Eating the right foods for fertility can increase a woman's libido and promote a healthy sex life.

CHAPTER 2

14-Day Meal Plan

DAY 1

Breakfast: Overnight Oats

Lunch: Salmon and kale Salad

Dinner: Salmon and Asparagus Quinoa Bowl

DAY 2

Breakfast: Chia Pudding

Lunch: Avocado Toast with Sprouts

Dinner: Lentil and Roasted Squash Salad

DAY 3

Breakfast: Egg Burrito

Lunch: Quinoa Bowl with Sweet Potatoes and Kale

Dinner: Garlic Encrusted Roast Chicken with Kale

DAY 4

Breakfast: Avocado Toast

Lunch: Greek Eggplant Stew

Dinner: Kale and Mushroom Frittata

DAY 5

Breakfast: Buckwheat Porridge

Lunch: Grilled Chicken and Vegetable Wrap

Dinner: Avocado and Quinoa Stuffed Roasted Red Peppers

DAY 6

Breakfast: Fertility Veggie Scramble

Lunch: Asparagus and Mushroom Frittata

Dinner: Lemon Roasted Shrimp & Veggie Bowl

DAY 7

Breakfast: Fertility Omelette

Lunch: Lentil Soup with Spinach and Cumin

Dinner: Spinach and Parmesan Stuffed Salmon

DAY 8

Breakfast: Poached Eggs with Asparagus

Lunch: Lentil Burgers with Grilled Zucchini

Dinner: Quinoa, Tomato & Pepper Salad

DAY 9

Breakfast: Sweet Potato Toast

Lunch: Turkey and Black Bean Chili

Dinner: Sweet Potato, Black Bean and Pesto Burgers

DAY 10

Breakfast: Salmon Hash with Spinach

Lunch: Roasted Sweet Potato and Kale Soup

Dinner: TunaStuffed Avocado with Walnut Crust

DAY 11

Breakfast: Overnight Oats

Lunch: Salmon and kale Salad

Dinner: Salmon and Asparagus Quinoa Bowl

DAY 12

Breakfast: Chia Pudding

Lunch: Avocado Toast with Sprouts

Dinner: Lentil and Roasted Squash Salad

DAY 13

Breakfast: Egg Burrito

Lunch: Quinoa Bowl with Sweet Potatoes and Kale

Dinner: Garlic Encrusted Roast Chicken with Kale

DAY 14

Breakfast: Avocado Toast

Lunch: Greek Eggplant Stew

Dinner: Kale and Mushroom Frittata

CHAPTER 3

30 Nutritious Recipes that's Boosts Fertility

BREAKFAST

Overnight Oats

Start your day off right with this nutrientpacked breakfast! It's packed with healthy carbohydrates and fiber which helps to support hormones in men and women with fertility issues.

Ingredients:

1/2 cup rolled oats

1/2 cup any milk of choice

1/2 cup yogurt

1/2 teaspoon ground cinnamon

1 tablespoon honey

1 tablespoon chia seeds

1/4 cup berries or sliced fruit

Preparation Time: 10 minutes

Method of Preparation:

1. In a small bowl, combine the oats, milk, yogurt, cinnamon, and honey.

2. Stir to combine and pour into a mason jar with a tightfitting lid.

3. Add the chia seeds and berries, stir, and seal the jar.

4. Refrigerate overnight or for at least 8 hours.

Serving suggestion: Serve with fresh berries and a handful of nuts for added texture and nutrients.

Chia Pudding

Give your health a nutritious boost with this chia pudding! Rich in fiber, protein, and omega3 fatty acids, this chia pudding can help those suffering from infertility by providing important nutrients to aid in conception.

Ingredients:

1/2 cup chia seeds

1 cup any milk of choice

1 teaspoon vanilla extract

1 tablespoon honey

1/4 cup berries or sliced fruit

Preparation Time: 10 minutes

Method of Preparation:

1. In a small bowl, stir together the chia seeds, milk, vanilla, and honey.

2. Pour the mixture into a mason jar with a tightfitting lid and stir.

3. Add the berries and stir.

4. Seal the jar and refrigerate for at least 8 hours or overnight.

Serving suggestion: Serve with fresh berries and a handful of nuts for added texture and nutrients.

Egg Burrito

Keep your energy levels up and your fertility in check with this tasty egg burrito! Packed with healthy protein and complex carbohydrates, this burrito provides longlasting energy and hormone support to those with fertility issues.

Ingredients:

3 large eggs

1/4 cup diced bell pepper

1/4 cup diced onion

1/4 cup grated cheese

2 tablespoons olive oil

Whole wheat or corn tortilla

Preparation Time: 10 minutes

Method of Preparation:

1. Heat the olive oil in a medium skillet over mediumhigh heat.

2. Add the bell pepper and onion and cook for 2 minutes, until softened.

3. Add the eggs and scramble until cooked.

4. Remove the pan from the heat and stir in the grated cheese.

5. Warm the tortillas, then spoon the egg mixture into each one.

6. Fold each side of the tortillas over the eggs and enjoy.

Serving suggestion: Serve with salsa and/or avocado slices for added flavor.

Avocado Toast

Upgrade your breakfast with this nutritious avocado toast! Rich in heart healthy fats, it can help optimize hormone levels in men and women struggling with fertility.

Ingredients:

1 ripe avocado

2 slices whole wheat bread

1/2 lime

Pinch of salt

Preparation Time: 5 minutes

Method of Preparation:

1. Toast the bread until golden brown.

2. While it's toasting, halve the avocado and scoop out the flesh into a bowl.

3. Mash with a fork until smooth, then squeeze in the juice of half a lime and season with a pinch of salt.

4. Spread the mashed avocado onto the toast, cut into triangles, and enjoy.

Serving suggestion: Serve this easy toast with a fried egg or boiled egg for added protein.

Buckwheat Porridge

Get the nutrition you need with this delicious porridge! Not only is it high in fiber and healthy carbohydrates, it also contains many essential vitamins and minerals which are critical for proper fertility health.

Ingredients:

1/2 cup buckwheat groats

1 cup milk of choice

1 teaspoon ground cinnamon

1 tablespoon honey

1/4 cup sliced or diced fruit

Preparation Time: 10 minutes

Method of Preparation:

1. In a small saucepan, bring the buckwheat groats and milk to a boil over medium heat.

2. Reduce the heat and simmer for 5 minutes, stirring occasionally.

3. Stir in the cinnamon and honey, then remove from the heat and let cool.

Serving suggestion: Add a dollop of yogurt or a drizzle of honey for added sweetness.

Fertility Veggie Scramble

Start your day off on the right foot with this nutritious scramble! Packed with essential vitamins and minerals, this scramble is ideal for those suffering from infertility to keep both their energy and fertility levels in check.

Ingredients:

3 eggs

1/4 cup diced bell pepper

1/4 cup diced onion

1/4 cup baby spinach

1 tablespoon olive oil

Preparation Time: 10 minutes

Method of Preparation:

1. Heat the olive oil in a medium skillet over mediumhigh heat.

2. Add the bell pepper and onion and cook for 2 minutes, until softened.

3. Add the eggs and scramble until cooked.

4. Add the spinach and cook until wilted.

5. Season with a pinch of salt and pepper if desired and remove from the heat.

Serving suggestion: Serve this scramble with a dollop of yogurt, a slice of toast, or a side of sweet potatoes.

Fertility Omelette

Get a healthy dose of protein and healthy fats to support reproductive health with this scrumptious omelette! Great for breakfast or brunch, the fertility omelette is a nourishing meal that helps support the body's natural hormone balance.

Ingredients:

3 eggs

1/4 cup diced bell pepper

1/4 cup diced onion

1/4 cup grated cheese

2 tablespoons olive oil

Preparation Time: 10 minutes

Method of Preparation:

1. Heat the olive oil in a medium skillet over mediumhigh heat.

2. Add the bell pepper and onion and cook for 2 minutes, until softened.

3. Whisk the eggs together and pour over the vegetables.

4. Stir gently until the eggs are set and then sprinkle with the grated cheese.

5. Fold one side of the omelette over and cook for 23 minutes until golden brown.

6. Carefully flip and cook for another 2 minutes.

7. Slide the omelette onto a plate and enjoy.

Serving suggestion: Serve this omelette with a side of toast and slices of avocado.

Poached Eggs with Asparagus

Love eggs and asparagus? Then this delicious meal is perfect for you! Packed with nutrientrich ingredients, poached eggs with asparagus provide essential vitamins, minerals, and healthy fats to support fertility in both men and women.

Ingredients:

4 eggs

1 bunch asparagus

1 tablespoon butter

2 tablespoons white vinegar

Pinch of salt

Preparation Time: 10 minutes

Method of Preparation:

1. Fill a medium saucepan with 2 inches of water and bring to a simmer.

2. Add the vinegar and a pinch of salt, then reduce the heat to low.

3. Melt the butter in a skillet over mediumhigh heat and add the asparagus.

4. Cook until tender, then remove from the heat and set aside.

5. Crack each egg into its own small bowl and carefully add the eggs to the simmering water.

6. Cook for 34 minutes, then carefully remove with a slotted spoon.

7. Divide the asparagus between two plates and top with the poached eggs.

8. Season with a pinch of salt and serve immediately.

Serving suggestion: Serve with a slice of toast for a complete meal.

Sweet Potato Toast

Upgrade your breakfast with this delectable sweet potato toast! Full of complex carbohydrates and dietary fiber, sweet potato toast can help provide important hormone balance for those struggling with infertility.

Ingredients:

2 sweet potatoes, thinly sliced

1 tablespoon olive oil

Pinch of salt

Optional toppings such as mashed avocado, sliced tomatoes, or cottage cheese

Preparation Time: 15 minutes

Method of Preparation:

1. Preheat the oven to 400°F.

2. Brush both sides of the sweet potato slices with olive oil and place in a single layer on a baking sheet.

3. Sprinkle with a pinch of salt.

4. Bake for 20-25 minutes, flipping once, until golden brown and tender.

5. Top each slice with desired toppings and enjoy.

Serving suggestion: Enjoy with a fried egg or boiled egg for added protein.

Salmon Hash with Spinach

Start your day off with this hearty and nourishing salmon hash! Rich in essential vitamins and minerals, it provides essential nutrition for those suffering from infertility and helps to support reproductive health.

Ingredients:

1 tablespoon olive oil

1 small onion, diced

2 cloves garlic, minced

2 cups cooked salmon chunks

2 cups diced sweet potatoes

1 cup frozen spinach

Pinch of salt and pepper

Optional toppings such as fresh herbs, hot sauce, or a dollop of yogurt

Preparation Time: 10 minutes

Method of Preparation:

1. Heat the olive oil in a large skillet over mediumhigh heat.

2. Add the onion and garlic and cook for 2 minutes until softened.

3. Add the salmon, sweet potatoes, and spinach and season with a pinch of salt and pepper.

4. Cook for 8-10 minutes until the sweet potatoes are tender.

5. Divide between two plates and top with desired toppings.

Serving suggestion: Serve this hash with a side of toast and a dollop of yogurt for added creaminess.

LUNCH

Salmon and Kale Salad

This delicious and nutritious salad combines healthy salmon with superfood kale, providing essential vitamins and minerals to help combat infertility.

Ingredients:

120g fresh salmon fillet

2 tablespoons olive oil

2 teaspoons fresh dill , chopped

2 handfuls baby kale leaves

2 tablespoons freshsqueezed lemon juice

1 teaspoon garlic powder

2 tablespoons feta cheese

1/4 teaspoon cracked black pepper

Preparation time: 15 minutes

Method of Preparation:

1. Preheat the oven to 400 degrees.

2. Place salmon on a baking sheet covered with parchment paper and season with dill, garlic powder, and cracked black pepper.

3. Drizzle olive oil over the salmon and roast in preheated oven for 10 minutes.

4. Meanwhile, add kale leaves to a large bowl and squeeze lemon juice on top. Massage the kale leaves and lemon juice together until the leaves are softened.

5. Once the salmon is cooked, flake it apart and add to the bowl of kale.

6. Sprinkle feta cheese over the salmon and kale and toss everything together.

Serving suggestion: Serve with whole wheat toast or quinoa for a complete meal.

Avocado Toast with Sprouts

Get a boost of nutrientrich food with this powerpacked combination of superfoods avocado and sprouts. It's an ideal meal for promote fertility and reproductive health.

Ingredients:

1 large avocado

2 slices of whole wheat bread, toasted

1 teaspoon olive oil

2 tablespoons fresh lemon juice

Salt and pepper, to taste

1/4 cup alfalfa sprouts

1/4 cup Parmesan cheese

Preparation time: 10 minutes

Method of Preparation:

1. Cut the avocado in half and remove the stone. Scoop out the flesh and mash it with a fork in a small bowl.

2. Drizzle olive oil and lemon juice over the mashed avocado and season with salt and pepper. Mix together until combined.

3. Spread the avocado mixture onto the toasted slices of bread and sprinkle the alfalfa sprouts and Parmesan cheese on top.

Serving suggestion: Enjoy the avocado toast with a simple side salad or a cup of soup.

Quinoa Bowl with Sweet Potatoes and Kale

Get a vitaminrich meal with this powerful combination of

quinoa, sweet potatoes, and kale. It has plenty of antioxidants to boost fertility and provide essential vitamins and minerals.

Ingredients:

1 cup cooked quinoa

1 large sweet potato, peeled and diced

2 tablespoons olive oil

1 teaspoon garlic powder

2 cups kale, stems removed and chopped

2 tablespoons freshlysqueezed lemon juice

Salt and pepper, to taste

1/4 cup finelychopped walnuts

Preparation time: 30 minutes

Method of Preparation:

1. Preheat the oven to 400 degrees.

2. Place the diced sweet potato on a baking sheet covered with parchment paper and drizzle with olive oil. Sprinkle

garlic powder over the potatoes and toss until evenly coated.

3. Bake in preheated oven for 20-25 minutes until golden and tender.

4. Meanwhile, add the kale to a large bowl and massage with the lemon juice until the leaves are softened.

5. In a large bowl, combine the cooked quinoa, roasted sweet potatoes, and kale. Sprinkle salt and pepper to taste.

Serving suggestion: Serve with a dollop of Greek yogurt for added creaminess.

Greek Eggplant Stew

This eggplant stew combines traditional spices with healthy vegetables, giving your body the nutrients it needs while also releasing powerful antioxidants.

Ingredients:

2 tablespoons olive oil

1 large onion, chopped

2 cloves garlic, minced

1 large eggplant, chopped

2 cans (14.5 ounces each) diced tomatoes

1 cup vegetable broth

1 teaspoon dried oregano

1 teaspoon dried basil

Salt and pepper, to taste

1/4 cup feta cheese

2 tablespoons freshly chopped parsley

Preparation time: 35 minutes

Method of Preparation:

1. Heat olive oil in a large saucepan over medium heat.

2. Add the onion and sauté for 5 minutes until softened.

3. Add the garlic and eggplant and sauté for 5 more minutes.

4. Add the diced tomatoes, vegetable broth, oregano, and basil. Bring to a simmer and cook for 20 minutes. Season with salt and pepper to taste.

Serving suggestion: Serve with brown rice or quinoa for a complete meal.

Grilled Chicken and Vegetable Wrap

This wrap fuses delicious grilled chicken with vibrant vegetables, providing a nutritionally balanced meal full of antioxidantrich ingredients to help support fertility.

Ingredients:

2 boneless, skinless chicken breasts

2 tablespoons olive oil

2 cloves garlic, minced

1/2 teaspoon paprika

2 large wraps

2 tablespoons Greek yogurt

1 large tomato, diced

1/2 small red onion, diced

2 cups baby spinach leaves

Preparation time: 25 minutes

Method of Preparation:

1. Preheat the grill to mediumhigh heat.

2. Drizzle olive oil over the chicken and season with garlic, paprika, salt, and pepper.

3. Grill the chicken on each side for 810 minutes until cooked through.

4. Meanwhile, spread the wraps on a flat surface. Spread the yogurt onto the wraps and top with the diced tomatoes, red onion, and baby spinach.

5. Once the chicken is cooked, thinly slice and top the wraps with the grilled chicken.

6. Roll up the wraps and serve.

Serving suggestion: Serve the wraps with a side of fresh fruit for a complete meal.

Asparagus and Mushroom Frittata

Start your day off with this savory, nutrientpacked frittata. It contains a wealth of antioxidants to help stimulate productive hormones in the body, aiding in fertility.

Ingredients:

2 tablespoons olive oil

1/2 onion, diced

1 clove garlic, minced

2 cups mushrooms, sliced

1 cup asparagus, cut into 1inch pieces

Salt and pepper, to taste

6 large eggs, lightly beaten

1/4 cup shredded mozzarella cheese

2 tablespoons freshly chopped parsley

Preparation time: 30 minutes

Method of Preparation:

1. Heat the olive oil in a large skillet over medium heat.

2. Add the onion and garlic and sauté for 5 minutes until softened.

3. Add the mushrooms and asparagus and sauté for an additional 5 minutes. Season with salt and pepper.

4. Pour the beaten eggs into the skillet and stir everything together.

5. Sprinkle the mozzarella cheese over the frittata and reduce the heat to low.

6. Cover the skillet and cook for 12-15 minutes until the frittata is set.

7. Sprinkle the freshlychopped parsley over the top. Serve warm.

Serving suggestion: Enjoy the frittata with a simple side salad for a complete meal.

Lentil Soup with Spinach and Cumin

Infertility sufferers can reap the goodness of lentil, spinach, and cumin in this nutritious, flavorful soup. It's packed with essential vitamins and minerals to help combat infertility.

Ingredients:

2 tablespoons olive oil

1/2 onion, minced

2 cloves garlic, minced

2 carrots, diced

2 celery stalks, diced

1 teaspoon ground cumin

1/4 teaspoon chili powder

2 cups vegetable broth

1 cup dry lentils, rinsed

1 can (14.5 ounces) diced tomatoes

2 cups baby spinach leaves

Salt and pepper, to taste

Preparation time: 45 minutes

Method of Preparation:

1. Heat the olive oil in a large pot over medium heat.

2. Add the onion, garlic, carrots, and celery. Sauté for 5 minutes until softened.

3. Add the cumin and chili powder and stir to combine.

4. Increase the heat to mediumhigh and add the vegetable broth, lentils, and diced tomatoes. Bring to a boil and reduce the heat to low. Simmer for 30 minutes.

5. Add the spinach leaves and season with salt and pepper. Simmer for an additional 5 minutes.

Serving suggestion: Enjoy the soup with a dollop of Greek yogurt and freshlychopped parsley.

Lentil Burgers with Grilled Zucchini

Get all the fertilitypromoting benefits of lentils with this savory and satisfying burger. It's topped with grilled zucchini and is full of essential nutrients to support reproductive health.

Ingredients:

1 cup dry lentils, rinsed

2 cloves garlic, minced

1 teaspoon ground cumin

1 teaspoon smoked paprika

2 tablespoons freshlychopped parsley

2 tablespoons quick oats

1/2 cup yellow onion, finely chopped

Salt and pepper, to taste

2 tablespoons olive oil

2 small zucchini, sliced

Preparation time: 30 minutes

Method of Preparation:

1. Preheat the oven to 375 degrees.

2. In a mediumsized bowl, combine the lentils, garlic, cumin, smoked paprika, parsley, oats, and onion. Season with salt and pepper to taste.

3. Form the mixture into 8 patties and place on a baking sheet lined with parchment paper.

4. Bake in preheated oven for 20 minutes.

5. Meanwhile, heat the olive oil in a large skillet over medium heat.

6. Add the zucchini slices and cook for 810 minutes until golden and tender.

Serving suggestion: Enjoy the burgers with a side salad or a simple green vegetable.

Turkey and Black Bean Chili

Make the most out of fertilitysupporting black beans with this flavorful chili. It combines turkey, black beans, and a host of spices, providing an ample amount of vitamins and minerals to support fertility.

Ingredients:

1 tablespoon olive oil

1/2 onion, diced

1 jalapeno pepper, finely chopped

4 cloves garlic, minced

1 teaspoon ground cumin

1 teaspoon chili powder

1 pound ground turkey

2 cans (14.5 ounces each) diced tomatoes

2 cans (15 ounces each) black beans, drained

1 cup vegetable broth

Salt and pepper, to taste

1/4 cup freshlychopped cilantro

Preparation time: 30 minutes

Method of Preparation:

1. Heat the olive oil in a large pot over medium heat.

2. Add the onion, jalapeno pepper, garlic, cumin, and chili powder. Sauté for 5 minutes until softened.

3. Add the ground turkey and cook, breaking up the meat with a wooden spoon, until the meat is no longer pink, about 8 minutes.

4. Add the diced tomatoes, black beans, and vegetable broth to the pot. Bring to a simmer and cook for 20 minutes.

5. Season with salt and pepper to taste.

Serving suggestion: Enjoy the chili with a side of brown rice or a simple side salad.

Roasted Sweet Potato and Kale Soup

Full of essential vitamins and minerals, this delicious soup is perfect for fertility health. It combines hearty sweet potatoes with powerhouse vegetables, like kale, to promote healthy reproductive hormones.

Ingredients:

2 tablespoons olive oil

1 large onion, diced

3 cloves garlic, minced

2 large sweet potatoes, peeled and diced

1 teaspoon ground cumin

1 teaspoon smoked paprika

2 cups vegetable broth

3 cups kale, stems removed and chopped

Salt and pepper, to taste

2 tablespoons freshlychopped parsley

Preparation time: 40 minutes

Method of Preparation:

1. Preheat the oven to 400 degrees.

2. Spread the diced sweet potatoes on a baking sheet lined with parchment paper and drizzle with 1 tablespoon of olive oil. Sprinkle cumin and smoked paprika over the potatoes and toss until evenly coated.

3. Roast the potatoes in preheated oven for 25 minutes until golden and tender.

4. Meanwhile, heat the remaining olive oil in a large pot over medium heat.

5. Add the onion and garlic and sauté for 5 minutes until softened.

6. Add the roasted sweet potatoes, vegetable broth, and kale to the pot. Bring to a simmer and cook for 10 minutes.

7. Season with salt and pepper to taste.

Serving suggestion: Enjoy the soup with whole wheat toast or crackers for a complete meal.

DINNER

Salmon and Asparagus Quinoa Bowl

This tasty bowl combines the nutritious benefits of

Wild caught salmon, asparagus and quinoa, all rich in fertility boosting antioxidants and vitamins.

Ingredients:

2 (4ounce) salmon fillets

2 tablespoons olive oil

Salt and pepper

2 cups quinoa

4 cups chicken or vegetable broth

1 bunch asparagus (trimmed and chopped)

3 tablespoons fresh lemon juice

Preparation Time: 30 minutes

Method of Preparation:

1. Preheat oven to 350°F.

2. Rub olive oil over the salmon and season with salt and pepper. Place on a baking sheet and roast for 15 minutes.

3. Bring the broth to a boil in a large pot. Once boiling, add quinoa and reduce to low heat. Cover and cook for 20-25 minutes, until liquid is absorbed.

4. Heat the remaining olive oil in a large pan over medium heat. Add asparagus and lemon juice, season with salt and pepper. Cook for 5 minutes.

5. Once finished cooking, fluff quinoa with a fork and divide evenly into 4 bowls. Top with roasted salmon and asparagus.

Serving Suggestion: Serve the Salmon and Asparagus Quinoa Bowl with a side of simple greens and a glass of lemon water.

Lentil and Roasted Squash Salad

Loaded with fiber, protein and iron, this lentil and squash salad is a great source of fertilitypromoting nutrition.

Ingredients:

2 cups cubed butternut squash

2 tablespoons olive oil

1/2 teaspoon garlic powder

1/2 teaspoon ground cinnamon

1/4 teaspoon nutmeg

1 1/2 cups cooked lentils

1/4 cup chopped basil

3 tablespoons balsamic vinegar

2 tablespoons honey

Preparation Time: 40 minutes

Method of Preparation:

1. Preheat oven to 400°F.

2. Place the squash cubes on a baking sheet and toss with olive oil, garlic powder, cinnamon and nutmeg.

3. Roast for about 30 minutes, stirring the squash cubes halfway through.

4. In a large bowl, combine lentils, basil, vinegar, honey and roasted squash cubes. Stir to combine.

Serving Suggestion: Enjoy the salad on its own or pair it with grilled chicken and a piece of warm pita bread.

Garlic Encrusted Roast Chicken with Kale

This ovenbaked dish provides the perfect combination of fertilitysupporting garlic, lean chicken and nutrient-packed kale.

Ingredients:

2 (4ounce) boneless skinless chicken breasts

4 tablespoons olive oil, divided

2 cloves garlic, minced

1/2 teaspoon smoked paprika

1/4 teaspoon cayenne pepper

1 teaspoon dried oregano

1/2 teaspoon salt

1/4 teaspoon black pepper

2 bunches kale, stemmed and roughly chopped

Preparation Time: 25 minutes

Method of Preparation:

1. Preheat oven to 400°F.

2. Place chicken breasts on a baking sheet and brush with 2 tablespoons of olive oil.

3. In a small bowl, mix garlic, smoked paprika, cayenne pepper, oregano, salt and pepper. Rub the seasoning mix over the chicken breasts.

4. Bake the chicken for 18 minutes, until cooked through.

5. Heat the remaining 2 tablespoons of olive oil in a large skillet over medium high heat. Add kale and cook for 57 minutes, until it starts to wilt.

Serving Suggestion: Serve the Garlic Encrusted Roast Chicken with Kale with a light side salad, such as avocado and tomato, and whole wheat pita bread.

Kale and Mushroom Frittata

Packed with protein, iron, Vitamin C and other fertility boosting trace minerals, this frittata provides all the essential nutrition to help support a healthy, fertile body.

Ingredients:

3 tablespoons olive oil

1/2 onion, chopped

1 clove garlic, minced

1/2 teaspoon salt

1/4 teaspoon black pepper

1 (8ounce) package cremini mushrooms

2 cups chopped kale

8 eggs

2 tablespoons heavy cream

Preparation Time: 30 minutes

Method of Preparation:

1. Preheat oven to 375°F.

2. Heat olive oil in a large skillet over medium heat. Add onion and garlic and cook for 5 minutes.

3. Season with salt and pepper and add mushrooms and kale. Cook until the vegetables are soft, about 7-10 minutes.

4. In a medium bowl, whisk together eggs, cream, and remaining salt and pepper.

5. Pour the egg mixture over the vegetables in the skillet and stir lightly to combine.

6. Bake in preheated oven for 20-25 minutes, until the eggs are set.

Serving Suggestion: Serve the Kale and Mushroom Frittata with a side of sliced avocado and creamy goat cheese.

Avocado and Quinoa Stuffed Roasted Red Peppers

Rich with fertility enhancing antioxidants, omega3 fatty acids and vitamins A, C and K, this delicious dish is sure to provide your body with a wide range of fertility supporting nutrition.

Ingredients:

4 large red peppers

2 tablespoons olive oil

1/2 cup quinoa

1 cup vegetable broth

1/2 cup black beans, rinsed and drained

1/2 cup corn

1 avocado, diced

1/4 cup chopped cilantro

1/4 cup chopped green onion

2 tablespoons freshly squeezed lime juice

Preparation Time: 45 minutes

Method of Preparation:

1. Preheat oven to 400°F.

2. Cut the peppers in half lengthwise and remove the seeds. Place the pepper halves on a baking sheet and brush with olive oil.

3. Roast the peppers in preheated oven for 20 minutes, until just tender.

4. In the meantime, bring the broth and quinoa to a boil in a small saucepan. Once boiling, reduce the heat to low and cover the pot. Cook for 15 minutes, until the liquid is absorbed.

5. In a large bowl, mix cooked quinoa, black beans, corn, avocado, cilantro, green onion, and lime juice.

6. Once done roasting, stuff the peppers with the quinoa mixture.

Serving Suggestion: Serve the peppers with a side of mixed greens or sautéed vegetables.

Lemon Roasted Shrimp & Veggie Bowl

A hearty, healthy bowl of fertilitysupporting shrimp, veggies and lemon boast a variety of vitamins and minerals, like zinc, that help promote a healthy uterus.

Ingredients:

1 pound shrimp, peeled and deveined

2 tablespoons olive oil

1 tablespoon crushed garlic

1 teaspoon smoked paprika

Juice of 1 lemon

1/2 teaspoon salt

1/4 teaspoon black pepper

2 cups broccoli florets

1 cup cubed butternut squash

1 cup cherry tomatoes, halved

Preparation Time: 25 minutes

Method of Preparation:

1. Preheat oven to 400°F.

2. In a medium bowl, mix shrimp, olive oil, garlic, smoked paprika, lemon juice, salt and pepper.

3. Spread the shrimp mixture on a baking sheet. Add the broccoli, squash, and tomatoes to the baking sheet.

4. Roast for 15-20 minutes, until the vegetables are soft and the shrimp are cooked through.

Serving Suggestion: Enjoy the Lemon Roasted Shrimp & Veggie Bowl with a side of brown rice or quinoa and a crisp side salad.

Spinach and Parmesan Stuffed Salmon

With a generous helping of zinc, omega3 fatty acids and fertility supporting antioxidants, this tasty Mediterranean style dish will help maximize your fertility potential.

Ingredients:

2 (4ounce) salmon fillets

2 tablespoons olive oil

Salt and pepper

2 cups fresh spinach

1/2 cup shredded Parmesan cheese

1/4 cup diced onion

1/4 cup diced red bell pepper

Preparation Time: 30 minutes

Method of Preparation:

1. Preheat oven to 350°F.

2. Rub olive oil over the salmon fillets and season with salt and pepper.

3. Place the salmon fillets in an ovensafe dish and set aside.

4. In a medium bowl, mix spinach, Parmesan cheese, onion, and red bell pepper.

5. Place the spinach mixture on top of the salmon fillets and bake for 18-20 minutes, until the salmon is cooked through.

Serving Suggestion: Enjoy the Spinach and Parmesan Stuffed Salmon with a side of roasted sweet potatoes and steamed kale.

Quinoa, Tomato & Pepper Salad

Loaded with nutrients known to support fertility like zinc and omega3 fatty acids, this quinoa salad provides a delicious, healthful boost for those looking to improve fertility.

Ingredients:

1 1/2 cups cooked quinoa

1/4 cup extravirgin olive oil

Juice of 1 lemon

1/2 teaspoon smoked paprika

1/4 teaspoon salt

1/2 teaspoon freshly ground black pepper

1 red bell pepper, diced

3 tomatoes, diced

1/2 cup feta cheese

2 tablespoons chopped dill

Preparation Time: 20 minutes

Method of Preparation:

1. In a small bowl, whisk together olive oil, lemon juice, smoked paprika, salt and pepper.

2. In a medium bowl, combine quinoa, bell pepper, tomatoes, feta cheese, and dill.

3. Drizzle the olive oil mixture over the quinoa mixture and stir to combine.

Serving Suggestion: Enjoy the Quinoa, Tomato & Pepper Salad on its own as a light meal or serve it with grilled chicken and a side of chickpeas.

Sweet Potato, Black Bean and Pesto Burgers

This fiber and protein packed burger provides essential fertility promoting vitamins and minerals like iron and folate.

Ingredients:

2 large sweet potatoes

1 tablespoon olive oil

1 (15ounce) can black beans, drained and rinsed

1/2 cup cooked quinoa

2 garlic cloves, minced

1/2 teaspoon ground cumin

1/2 teaspoon chili powder

1/4 teaspoon salt

1/4 cup pesto sauce

Preparation Time: 30 minutes

Method of Preparation:

1. Preheat oven to 400°F.

2. Pierce the sweet potatoes with a fork a few times and bake for 3035 minutes, until they are tender.

3. Once the potatoes have cooled, peel the skins and mash the sweet potatoes in a medium bowl.

4. Add beans, quinoa, garlic, cumin, chili powder, and salt to the mashed sweet potatoes and mix until everything is combined.

5. Form the mixture into patties and place on a baking sheet. Bake for 20-25 minutes, until the burgers are lightly browned.

Serving Suggestion: Enjoy the Sweet Potato, Black Bean and Pesto Burgers on a whole wheat bun with lettuce, tomato and a side of homemade sweet potato fries.

Tuna Stuffed Avocado with Walnut Crust

A delicious and nutrient dense dish, this tuna-stuffed avocado is a great source of omega3 fatty acids, fertility boosting vitamins and minerals like zinc and selenium.

Ingredients:

2 (5ounce) cans tuna, drained

1 tablespoon mayonnaise

2 tablespoons diced celery

2 tablespoons diced red onion

1 tablespoon freshly squeezed lemon juice

2 avocados, halved and pitted

2 tablespoons breadcrumbs

2 tablespoons finely chopped walnuts

Preparation Time: 15 minutes

Method of Preparation:

1. In a medium bowl, mix tuna, mayonnaise, celery, red onion, and lemon juice until everything is combined.

2. Scoop a portion of the tuna mixture into the center of each avocado half.

3. In a small bowl, mix breadcrumbs and walnuts.

4. Sprinkle the walnut breadcrumb mixture over each tuna-stuffed avocado.

5. Place the avocados on a baking sheet and bake for 10 minutes, until lightly browned.

Serving Suggestion: Enjoy the tuna-stuffed Avocado with Walnut Crust with a side of steamed broccoli and brown rice.

CONCLUSION

Millions of women across the globe are dealing with infertility, so stay hopeful and know that there are solutions available.

Keep the focus on the positive and obtain advice from an expert.

The information in this book should have given you insight into fertility treatments and nutrition.

Although it can be a difficult path, you don't have to go it alone.

For emotional support, reach out to family and friends or connect with other people facing similar struggles.

Additionally, if needed, don't hesitate to contact a mental health specialist.

Make sure to discuss fertility treatments and expectations with your partner.

Everyone's journeys will be different, so it's okay if you want different solutions.